¡EMERGENCIA!
Emergency Translation Manual

Emergency Caregivers Guide
to Communication with Spanish Speakers

Lisa Maitland de Hernández, EMT-A

D0154669

DELMAR

THOMSON LEARNING

Australia Canada Mexico Singapore Spain United Kingdom United States

DELMAR

THOMSON LEARNING

¡Emergencia!
Emergency Translation Manual
by
Lisa Maitland de Hernández

Health Care Publishing Director:
William Brottmiller

Executive Editor:
Cathy L. Esperti

Editorial Assistant:
Matt Thouin

Executive Marketing Manager:
Dawn F. Gerrain

Channel Manager:
Jennifer McAvey

Art/Design Coordinator:
Mary Colleen Liburdi

Table of Contents

Preface

As emergency caregivers, we interact daily with a diverse population. Part of the key to providing quality care is communication. As communities diversify, the need to communicate in languages other than English becomes a necessity.

Emergencia will not teach the Spanish language, but will provide the questions necessary to elicit specific care-related answers from Spanish-speaking patients. Most questions are phrased so that the responses required are either "yes" or "no". Thus, it is not necessary to spend valuable time looking for translations of the responses.

Before using *Emergencia*, become familiar with the manual. The English questions are found on the left-hand side of each page. Their Spanish counterparts and phonetic pronunciations are on the right. Become familiar with the commonly used phrases and body parts. Try to "sound out" the phonetic pronunciations next to the Spanish phrases before you actually have to use them.

At the beginning of each chapter, you will find questions that may be needed on an ongoing basis. Having these handy will prevent the constant need to page back and forth between sections. These phrases are somewhat different depending on the emergency.

The manual has tabbed sections relating to: medical emergencies, trauma, childbirth, allergic reactions, and other areas. Therefore, it is not necessary to go through the entire manual when presented with a specific ailment or injury.

The questions within each section will begin broadly and become more specific. This will allow you to rule out one diagnosis and quickly move on to the next possibility.

Emergencia was written to make your job easier, not more difficult. If you find that showing rather than speaking a question is more beneficial, do it! However you are able to communicate with someone in need, it will always lead to a higher quality of care.

Acknowledgements

Reviewers

The reviewers of *Emergencia* provided numerous suggestions and improvements for the manual. Their wealth of practical experience and knowledge was of great help when developing the manual for use in the field. I would like to thank them for their insights, input, time and commitment to quality. Both are amazing to watch in action and work beside. Thank you.

Ken Brown, NREMT-P

Captain William C. Rosier—Howard County, Maryland Department of Fire & Rescue Services

Thanks must also be extended to my friend Dwight A. Polk, MSW, NREMT-P for his encouragement to move forward, and the contacts to make this project finally come to fruition. Thank you.

Language Advisor

Often language can be a difficult thing. While many translations in the manual are fairly simple, some required translations that Spanish speakers from many countries, using different words for the same things, would understand. The translations took quite a few arduous hours to complete, and without the review of a native Spanish speaker, this project might have proven to be less than effective. To my friend, advisor, husband, and chief cheerleader, José A. Hernández, I wish to express my gratitude and heartfelt thanks for the late hours, endless patience, and belief in me. ¡Gracias por todo!

Finally, I would also like to thank the many firefighters, officers, EMTs, CRTs and EMT-Ps with whom I have had the privilege of working. It was with them the idea for this manual was born.

Dedication

For my sons Liam Alejandro and Aidan Emmanuel
You are the reasons I endeavor to be, do, and learn more.

List of Figures

Chapter 1
Common Words and Phrases

Common Words

Colors	Colores	*[Coe-lore-ace]*
Red	Rojo	*[roe-hoe]*
Green	Verde	*[vare-day]*
Blue	Azul	*[ah-zool]*
Black	Negro	*[nay-grow]*
Yellow	Amarillo	*[ah-mar-ee-yo]*
Brown	Café	*[cah-fay]*
White	Blanco	*[blahn-coe]*
Gray	Gris	*[grease]*

Numbers	Numeros	*[New-mare-ohs]*
1	Uno	*[ew-no]*
2	Dos	*[dose]*
3	Tres	*[trace]*
4	Cuatro	*[kwa-troe]*
5	Cinco	*[sink-oh]*
6	Seis	*[sace]*
7	Siete	*[see-eh-tay]*
8	Ocho	*[oh-choe]*
9	Nueve	*[new-ay-vay]*
10	Diez	*[dee-ace]*
20	Veinte	*[vehn-tay]*
30	Treinta	*[train-tah]*
40	Cuarenta	*[kwa-rent-ah]*
50	Cincuenta	*[sing-quent-ah]*
60	Seisenta	*[say-cent-ah]*
100	Cien	*[see-ehn]*

WORDS/PHRASES

References to Time of Day	Referencias a las Horas del Dìa	[Ray-feh-rehn-see-ahs ah llahs or-ahs dell Dee-ah]
Today	Hoy	[oy]
Yesterday	Ayer	[ah-yare]
Tomorrow	Mañana	[mahn-yahn-nah]
In the morning	Por la mañana	[pore lah mahn-yahn-nah]
In the afternoon	Por la tarde	[pore lah tar-day]
In the evening	Por la noche	[pore lah noe-chay]
Yesterday morning	Ayer por la mañana	[ah-yare pore lah mahn-yahn-nah]
Yesterday afternoon	Ayer por la tarde	[ah-yare pore lah tar-day]
Last night	Anoche	[ah-noe-chay]
Last week	Semana pasada	[say-mah-nah pah-sah-dah]
Last month	Mes pasado	[Mace pah-sah-doe]
Last year	Año pasado	[ahn-yoe pah-sah-doe]

Days of the Week	Dìas de la Semana	[Dee-ahs day lah Say-mah-nah]
Week	semana	[say-mah-nah]
Monday	lunes	[lew-nace]
Tuesday	martes	[mahr-tace]
Wednesday	miércoles	[mee-air-coe-lace]
Thursday	jueves	[who-ay-vace]
Friday	viernes	[vee-air-nace]
Saturday	sábado	[sah-bah-doe]
Sunday	domingo	[doe-meen-goe]

Year	Año	*[Ahn-yoh]*
January	enero	*[eh-neh-roe]*
February	febrero	*[feh-breh-roe]*
March	marzo	*[mahr-(t)zoe]*
April	abril	*[ah-breel]*
May	mayo	*[my-oh]*
June	junio	*[who-nee-oh]*
July	julio	*[who-lee-oh]*
August	agosto	*[ah-goe-stoe]*
September	septiembre	*[sep-tee-ehm-bray]*
October	octubre	*[oak-two-bray]*
November	noviembre	*[noe-vee-ehm-bray]*
December	diciembre	*[dee-see-ehm-bray]*

Who, What, When, Where, Why, How

Who	Quién	*[key-ehn]*
What	Qué	*[kay]*
When	Cuándo	*[kwan-doe]*
Where	Dónde	*[don-day]*
Why	Porqué	*[pour-kay]*
How	Cómo	*[coe-moe]*
How long	Por cuánto tiempo	*[pour kwahn-toe tee-ehm-poe]*
How many	Cuántos	*[kwan-toes]*

Direction	Dirección	*[Dee-wreck-see-own]*
Up	Arriba	*[ah-ree-bah]*
Down	Abajo	*[ah-bah-hoe]*
Left	Izquierda	*[eez-key-air-dah]*
Right	Derecho	*[dare-etch-oh]*

Direction	Dirección	*[Dee-wreck-see-own]*
Front	Delantero	*[day-lan-tare-oh]*
Back	Trasero	*[trah-sare-oh]*
Top	Encima	*[ehn-see-mah]*
Bottom	Abajo	*[ah-bah-hoe]*

Common Phrases

Important Phrases & Questions	Frases y Preguntas Importantes *[Frah-sace ee pray-goon-tahs eem-pore-tahn-tace]*
Hello, my name is _____.	Hola, me llamo _____. *[oh-lah, may yah-moe]*
I am a paramedic.	Soy un paramedico. *[soy oon pah-rah-meh-dee-coe]*
We are here to help you.	Estamos aquí para ayudarle. *[eh-stah-moes ak-key pah-rah-eye-you-dar-lay]*
Your name?	¿Su nombre? *[sue nom-bray]*
I do not speak Spanish well.	No hablo español bien. *[no ah-bloe eh-span-yole bee-ehn.]*
Do you speak English?	¿Habla inglés? *[ah-blah een-glaze]*
Does anyone here speak English?	¿Alguien aquí habla inglés? *[all-geeh-ehn ah-key ah-blah een-glaze]*
How old are you?	¿Cuántos años tiene? *[kwan-toes ahn-yoes tee-ehn-ay]*
Your birth date?	¿Su fecha de nacimiento? *[sue fetch-ah day nah-see me-ehn-toe]*
Your address?	¿Su dirección? *[sue-dee-wreck-see own]*

WORDS/PHRASES

Other helpful phrases	Otros frases	
Calm down.	Calmese.	*[call-may-say]*
It's okay.	Está bien.	*[eh-stah bee-ehn]*
Please speak slowly.	Hable despacio, por favor.	*[ah-blay dess-pahs-ee-oh pore-fah-wore]*
Please repeat.	Repita, por favor.	*[ray-pee-tah pore-fah-vore]*

People   Gente   *[Hen-tay]*

Who is this person, your...?	¿Quién es, su...?	*[key-ehn es, sue...]*
Where is your...?	¿Dónde está su...?	*[dohn-day es-tah sue...]*
Father	Padre	*[pah-dray]*
Mother	Madre	*[mah-dray]*
Husband	Esposo	*[eh-spoe-so]*
Wife	Esposa	*[eh-spoe-sah]*
Brother	Hermano	*[air-mah-no]*
Sister	Hermana	*[air-mah-nah]*
Child (male, female)	Hijo, Hija	*[ee-hoe, ee-hah]*
Grandfather	Abuelo	*[ah-bway-low]*
Grandmother	Abuela	*[ah-bway-lah]*
Uncle	Tío	*[tee-oh]*
Aunt	Tía	*[tee-ah]*
Cousin (male, female)	Primo, Prima	*[pree-moe, pree-mah]*
Friend (male, female)	Amigo, Amiga	*[ah-mee-go, ah-mee-gah]*
What is his/her name?	¿Cómo se llama?	*[coe-moe say yah-mah]*

Pronouns

Pronouns	Pronombres	[pro-nom-brays]
I / Me	Yo / Mi	[yo / me]
You	Usted	[oo-sted]
He	Él	[el]
She	Ella	[ay-yah]
We	Nosotros	[no-so-troes]
You (plural)	Ustedes	[oo-sted-ehs]
They	Ellos	[ay-yoes]

Chapter 2
The Body

The Head

Head	Cabeza	*[ka-bay-say]*
Eye(s)	Ojo(s)	*[oh-hoe]*
Ear(s)	Oreja(s)	*[or-ay-hah]*
Mouth	Boca	*[boe-kah]*
Tooth	Diente(s)	*[dee-ehn-tay]*
Tongue	Lengua	*[len-gwah]*
Lips	Labios	*[lah-bee-ohs]*
Hair	Pelo	*[pay-low]*
Forehead	Frente	*[fren-tay]*
Cheek	Mejilla	*[may-hee-ah]*
Nose	Nariz	*[nar-eez]*
Chin	Menton	*[men-tone]*
Throat	Garganta	*[gar-gan-tah]*

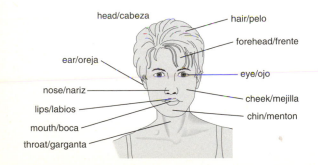

mouth/boca

lips/labios

teeth/dientes

tongue/lengua

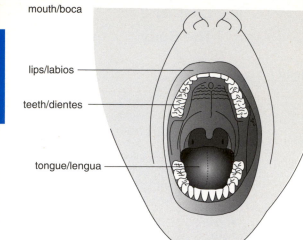

The Body - Inside

Brain	Cerebro	*[say-ray-bro]*
Heart	Corazon	*[core-ah-sewn]*
Lungs	Pulmones	*[pool-moan-ehs]*
Ribs	Costillas	*[coe-stee-yahs]*
Spine	Espina	*[eh-spee-nah]*
Stomach	Estómago	*[ehs-toe-mah-go]*
Liver	Hígado	*[ee-gah-doe]*
Kidneys	Riñones	*[reen-yone-ehs]*
Appendix	Apendice	*[ah-pen-dee-say]*
Bladder	Vejiga	*[vay-hee-gah]*
Rectum	Recto	*[wreck-toe]*

The Body - Inside

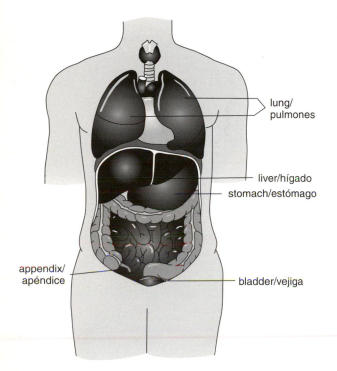

lung/
pulmones

liver/hígado

stomach/estómago

appendix/
apéndice

bladder/vejiga

The Body - Inside

Heart/Corazón

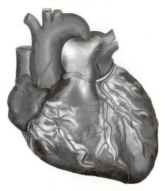

Brain/Cerebro

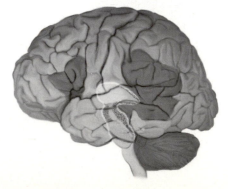

The Body - Inside

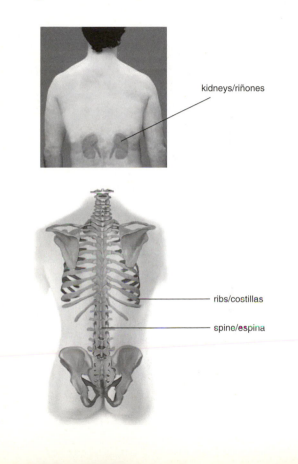

kidneys/riñones

ribs/costillas

spine/espina

The Body - Inside

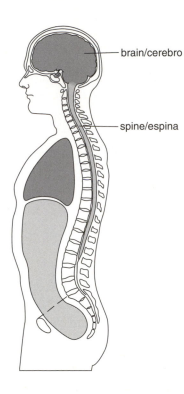

brain/cerebro

spine/espina

The Body - Inside

rectum/recto

The Body - Outside

English	Spanish	Pronunciation
Body	Cuerpo	*[kware-poe]*
Shoulder	Hombro	*[om-bro]*
Chest	Pecho	*[petch-oh]*
Elbow	Codo	*[coe-doe]*
Stomach	Estómago	*[ehs-tom-ago]*
Hip	Cadera	*[cah-dare-ah]*
Leg(s)	Pierna(s)	*[pee-air-nah(s)]*
Foot (Feet)	Pie(s)	*[pee-ay(s)]*
Toes	Dedos del Pie	*[day-does del pee-ay]*
Ankle	Tobillo	*[toe-bee-yo]*
Knee	Rodilla	*[row-dee-ya]*
Hand	Mano	*[mah-no]*
Fingers	Dedos de la mano	*[day-does de lah mah-no]*
Wrist	Muñeca	*[moon-yecka]*
Arm	Brazo	*[bra-soh]*
Back	Espalda	*[es-pal-dah]*
Neck	Cuello	*[kway-yo]*
Head	Cabeza	*[kah-bay-sah]*

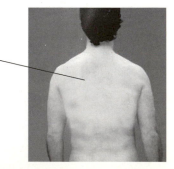

back/espalda

The Body - Outside

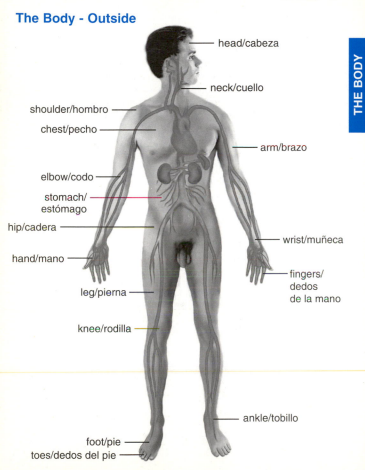

head/cabeza

neck/cuello

shoulder/hombro

chest/pecho

arm/brazo

elbow/codo

stomach/
estómago

hip/cadera

wrist/muñeca

hand/mano

fingers/
dedos
de la mano

leg/pierna

knee/rodilla

ankle/tobillo

foot/pie

toes/dedos del pie

Reproductive Organs

Penis	Pene	*[pen-ay]*
Testicles	Testículos	*[tehs-tee-coo-lows]*
Vagina	Vagina	*[vah-hee-nah]*
Uterus	Útero	*[oo-tare-oh]*
Ovary	Ovario	*[oh-vah-ree-oh]*
Breast	Pecho	*[petch-oh]*

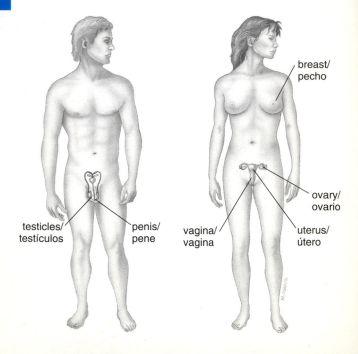

breast/
pecho

ovary/
ovario

testicles/
testículos

penis/
pene

vagina/
vagina

uterus/
útero

Chapter 3
Chest Pain

Are you hurt?	¿Está herido?	*[eh-tah air-ee-doe]*
Where?	¿Donde?	*[don-day]*
Show me.	Muéstreme.	*[mwhe-stray may]*
Did you faint?	¿Se desmayó?	*[say des-my-oh]*
Do you take any medications?	¿Toma medicinas?	*[toe-mah meh-dee-see-nahs]*
Get it.	Consíguelo	*[con-see-gay-low]*
Can you sit up?	¿Puede sentarse?	*[pway-day sen-tar-say]*
Please lie down.	Acuéstese, por favor.	*[ah-ques-tay-say poor fah-vore]*

Heart	**Corazon**	***[Core-ah-sewn]***
Heart Attack	Ataque del corazón	*[ah-tack-ay del core-ah-sewn]*
Where is the pain?	¿Dónde le duele?	*[don-day lay dway-lay]*
Chest	Pecho	*[petch-oh]*
Shoulder	Hombro	*[ohm-bro]*
Arm	Brazo	*[bra-soh]*
Neck	Cuello	*[kway-yo]*
Jaw	Mandíbula	*[mahn-dee-boo-lah]*
How long have you had the pain?	¿Por cuánto tiempo ha tenido ese dolor?	*[pour kwan-toe tee-em-poe ah ten-nee-doe eh-say doe-lore]*
Minutes?	¿Minutos?	*[me-new-toes]*
Hours?	¿Horas?	*[ore-ahs]*

CHEST PAIN

Heart	Corazon	[Core-ah-sewn]
Is the pain better when you rest?	¿El dolor es menos, cuando no se mueve?	[el doe-lore es may-knows, kwan-doe no say mway-vay]
From 1 to 10 (one is least, 10 is worst), how bad is the pain?	Uno a diez (uno es el menor, diez es el peor), el dolor es como?	[ew-no ah dee-ace (ew-no es el may-nor, dee-ace es el pay-ore), el doe-lore es coe-moe]
Is the pain sharp? throbbing?	¿El dolor es agudo? palpitando?	[el doe-lore es ah-goo-doe? pal-pee-tahn-doe?]
Do you feel pressure? tightness?	¿Se siente presión? apretado?	[say see-en-tay press-see-own? ah-pray-tah-doe?]
Do you sweat with the pain?	¿Suda con el dolor?	[sue-dah con el doe-lore]
Have you had this pain before?	¿Ha tenido este dolor anterior?	[ah ten-ee-doe eh-stay doe-lore ahn-tee-ree-ore]
Do you take medicine?	¿Toma medicina?	[toe-mah may-dee-see-nah]
Have you taken any today?	¿Lo ha tomado hoy?	[low ah toe-mah-doe oy]
How many?	¿Cuántos?	[kwan-toes]
When?	¿Cuándo?	[kwan-doe]
Minutes?	¿Minutos?	[me-new-toes]
Hours?	¿Horas?	[ore-ahs]

Questions for bystanders with an unconscious patient.

Did you see this person pass out?	¿Vió esta persona desmayarse?	*[vee-yo eh-stah pair-sew-nah des-my-are-say]*
How long ago?	¿Hace cuánto tiempo?	*[ah-say kwan-toe tee-em-poe]*
Minutes?	¿Minutos?	*[me-new-toes]*

Chapter 4
Gastro-Intestinal

Are you hurt?	¿Está herido?	[eh-tah air-ee-doe]
Where?	¿Dónde?	[don-day]
Show me.	Muéstreme.	[mwhe-stray may]
Did you faint?	¿Se desmayó?	[say des-my-oh]
Do you take any medications?	¿Toma medicinas?	[toe-mah meh-dee-see-nahs]
Get it.	Consíguelo.	[con-see-gay-low]
Can you sit up?	¿Puede sentarse?	[pway-day sen-tar-say]
Please lie down.	Acuéstese, por favor.	[ah-ques-tay-say poor fah-vore]

Gastro-Intestinal

Where is the pain?	¿Dónde está el dolor?	[don-day es-tah el doe-lore]
Is it sharp?	¿El dolor es agudo?	[el doe-lore es ah-goo-doe]
Does it ache?	¿Está adolorido?	[es-tah ah-doe-low-ree-doe]
When did it start?	¿Cuándo empezó?	[kwahn-doe em-peh-so]
Minutes?	¿Minutos?	[me-knew-toes]
Hours?	¿Horas?	[ore-ahs]
Days?	¿Días?	[dee-ahs]
When did you eat?	¿A qué hora comió la última?	[kwahn-doe coe-last mee-oh]
Breakfast	¿Desayuna?	[des-eye-oo-nah]
Lunch	¿Almuerzo?	[al-mwhere-so]
Dinner	¿Cena?	[sane-ah]

What did you eat?	¿Qué comió?	*[kay coe-mee-oh]*
Have you vomited?	¿Vomitó?	*[voe-mee-toe]*
What color was it?	¿El color del vómito?	*[el coe-lore del voe-mee-toe]*
Was there any blood?	¿Había sangre?	*[ah-bee-ah sahn-gray]*
Have you had diarrhea?	¿Ha tenido diarrea?	*[ah teh-nee-doe dee-ah-ray-ah]*
Constipation?	¿Ha tenido estreñimiento?	*[ah teh-nee-doe es-train-yee-mee-en-toe]*
Was there any blood?	¿Había sangre?	*[ah-bee-ah sahn-gray]*
Is there blood in your urine?	¿Hay sangre en su orina?	*[eye sahn-gray en sue Ore-ee-nah]*
Is there blood in your feces?	¿Hay sangre en su escremento?	*[eye sahn-gray en sue ehs-cray-men-toe]*
Are they...	¿Son...	*[sawn...]*
Yellow?	Amarillo?	*[ah-mar-ee-yo]*
Brown?	Café?	*[cah-fay]*
Black?	Negro?	*[nay-grow]*

Chapter 5
Respiratory

Are you hurt?	¿Está herido?	*[ehs-tah air-ee-doe]*
Where?	¿Donde?	*[don-day]*
Show me.	Muéstreme.	*[mwhe-stray may]*
Did you faint?	¿Se desmayó?	*[say des-my-oh]*
Do you take any medications?	¿Toma medicinas?	*[toe-mah meh-dee-see nahs]*
Get it.	Consíguelo.	*[con-see-gay-low]*
Can you sit up?	¿Puede sentarse?	*[pway-day sen-tar-say]*
Please lie down.	Acuéstese, por favor.	*[ah-ques-tay-say poor fah-vore]*

Lung	Pulmones	*[Pool-moan-ehs]*
Are you having trouble breathing?	¿No puede respirar?	*[no pway-day res-pee rar]*
Is something stuck in your throat?	¿Algo está en su garganta?	*[al-go estah en sue gar-gan-tah]*
Take a deep breath	Respire profundo.	*[reh-spee-ray pro-foon-doe]*
Breath.	Respire.	*[reh-spee-ray]*
Cough.	Tos.	*[tose]*
Do you smoke?	¿Fuma?	*[foo-mah]*
Do you have emphysema?	¿Tiene enfisema?	*[tee-eh-nay ehn-fee-say-mah?]*
Do you have allergies?	¿Tiene alergias?	*[tee-eh-nay ah-lare-hee-ahs]*

Asthma	Asma	[As-mah]

Do you have asthma?	¿Tiene asma?	[tee-eh-nay as-mah]
Do you use an inhaler?	¿Usa un inhalador?	[ooh-sah oon een-ha-lah-door]
Where is it?	¿Donde está?	[don-day es-tah]
Show me.	Muéstreme.	[mweh-stray-may]
Get it.	Consíguelo.	[con-see-gay-low]
Have you used it?	¿Lo usó?	[low ooh-sew]
Minutes?	¿Minutos?	[me-knew-toes]
Hours?	¿Horas?	[ore-ahs]
Do you take other medicine for asthma?	¿Toma otra medicina para asma?	[toe-mah oh-trah may-dee-see-nah pah-rah as-mah]
Where is it?	¿Dónde está?	[don-day es-tah]
Show me.	Muéstreme.	[mweh-stray-may]
Get it.	Consíguelo.	[con-see-gay-low]
Have you used it?	¿Lo usó?	[low ooh-sew]
Minutes?	¿Minutos?	[me-knew-toes]
Hours?	¿Horas?	[ore-ahs]
Do you have a cough?	¿Tiene tos?	[tee-eh-nay tose]
Do you have chest pain?	¿Tiene dolor en su pecho?	[tee-eh-nah doe-lore ehn sue petch-oh]
Does it hurt to take a deep breath?	¿Le duele a respirar profundo?	[lay dwell-lay ah ray-spee-rar Pro-foo-doe]
Do you have a fever?	¿Tiene fiebre?	[tee-eh-nay fee-eh-bray]
Do you have nausea or vomitng?	¿Tiene náusea o vómito?	[tee-eh-nay now-say-ah oh voe-mee-toe]

RESPIRATORY

Chapter 6
Seizures

English	Spanish	Pronunciation
Are you hurt?	¿Está herido?	[ehs-tah air-ee-doe]
Where?	¿Donde?	[don-day]
Show me.	Muéstreme.	[mwhe-stray may]
Did you faint?	¿Se desmayó?	[say des-my-oh]
Do you take any medications?	¿Toma medicinas?	[toe-mah meh-dee-see-nahs]
Get it.	Consíguelo.	[con-see-gay-low]
Can you sit up?	¿Puede sentarse?	[pway-day sen-tar-say]
Please lie down.	Acuéstese, por favor.	[ah-ques-tay-say poor fah-vore]

Seizures	Convulsiones	[Cone-vool-see-oh-nays]
To family/ bystanders	*A la familia/ asistentes*	
When did this happen?	¿Cuando le occurió?	[kwahn-doe lay oh-coo-ree-oh]
How long did it last?	¿Por cuanto le duró el ataque ?	[pour kwahn-toe lay do-roe el ah-tah-kay]
Has (s)he had more than one [seizure]?	¿Ha tenido más de uno?	[ah ten-ee-doe moss day ewe-no]
Does (s)he have epilepsy?	¿Tiene epilepsia?	[tee-en-nay eh-pee-lep see-ah]
Does (s)he take medicine for it?	¿Toma medicina para ese?	[toe-mah may-dee-see-nah par-ah eh-say]
Has (s)he taken it today?	¿La ha tomado hoy?	[la ah toe-mah-doe oy]

Seizures	Convulsiones	*[Cone-vool-see-oh-nays]*
Has (s)he had a high fever	¿Tenía una fiebre alta?	*[ten-ee-ah oo-nah fee-eh-bray al-tah]*
What temperature?	¿Qué temperatura?	*[kay tem-pare-ah-too-rah]*
For how long?	¿Por cuanto tiempo?	*[pour kwahn-toe tee-em-poe]*
Hours?	¿Horas?	*[ora-ahs]*
Days?	¿Días?	*[dee-ahs]*
Has (s)he had a brain injury?	¿Ha tenido un daño al cerebro?	*[ah ten-ee-doe oon don-yo all say-ray-bro]*
Did (s)he fall?	¿Se cayó?	*[say kai-yo]*

Chapter 7
Diabetes

English	Spanish	Pronunciation
Are you hurt?	¿Está herido?	*[ehs-tah air-ee-doe]*
Where?	¿Donde?	*[don-day]*
Show me.	Muéstreme.	*[mwhe-stray may]*
Did you faint?	¿Se desmayó?	*[say des-my-oh]*
Do you take any medications?	¿Toma medicinas?	*[toe-mah meh-dee-see-nahs]*
Get it.	Consíguelo.	*[con-see-gay-low]*
Can you sit up?	¿Puede sentarse?	*[pway-day sen-tar-say]*
Please lie down.	Acuéstese, por favor.	*[ah-ques-tay-say poor fah-vore]*

Diabetes — Diabetes

Do you have diabetes?	¿Tiene diabetes?	*[tee-en-nay dee-ah-beh-tays]*
Do you take insulin?	¿Toma insulina?	*[toe-mah een-sue-leen-ah]*
When did you take it?	¿Cuando lo tomó?	*[kwahn-doe low toe-moe]*
Today?	¿Hoy?	*[oy]*
Hours?	¿Horas?	*[ore-ahs]*
Minutes?	¿Minutos?	*[me-new-toes]*
Did you take too much?	¿Tomó demasiado?	*[toe-moe deh-mas-see-ah-doe]*
Have you eaten?	¿Comió?	*[coe-me-oh]*
When did you last eat?	¿Cuando comió?	*[kwahn-doe coe-me-oh]*
Breakfast	Desayuno	*[deh-sigh-ooh-no]*
Lunch	Almuerzo	*[al-mwhere-so]*
Dinner	Cena	*[say-nah]*

Diabetes

Diabetes	Diabetes	
Did you eat...	¿Comió...	*[coe-me-oh]*
Too much?	¿Demasiado?	*[deh-mah-see-ah-doe]*
Not enough?	¿Bastante?	*[bah-stahn-tay]*
Did you exercise too much?	¿Hace demasiado ejercicio?	*[ah-say deh-mah-see-ah-doe eh-hair- see-see-oh]*
When did the ____ start?	¿Cuando empezó el____?	*[kwahn-doe ehm-peh-so el____]*
dizziness	vertignoso	*[vare-teen-yo-so]*
weakness	debilidad	*[day-bee-lee-dod]*
headache	dolor de cabeza	*[doe-lore day cah-bay-sah]*
Today?	¿Hoy?	*[oy]*
Hours?	¿Horas?	*[ore-ahs]*
Minutes?	¿Minutos?	*[me-new-toes]*
Do you have pain in the abdomen?	¿Tiene dolor en su abdomen?	*[tee-en-nay doe-lore en sue ahb-doe-men]*
Have you vomited?	¿Vomitó?	*[voe-me-toe]*
Is your mouth dry?	¿Su boca está seca?	*[sue boe-cah es-tah seh-cah]*
Are you thirsty?	¿Tiene sed?	*[tee-en-nay said]*
hungry?	¿Tiene hambre?	*tee-en-nay ahm-bray?]*
Are you dizzy?	¿Está vertiginoso?	*[eh-stah vare-teen-yo-so]*
Do you have a headache?	¿Tiene dolor en su cabeza?	*[tee-en-nay doe-lore en sue cah-bay-sah]*
Do you have any...	¿Tiene...	*[tee-en-nay]*
candy	dulces	*[dool-says]*
orange juice	jugo de naranja	*[who-go day nah-rahn ha]*
sugar	azucar	*[ah-sue-car]*
Get it.	Consíguelo.	*[con-see-gay-low]*
Eat it.	Cómelo.	*[coe-may-low]*
Drink it.	Bébelo.	*[bay-bay-low]*

DIABETES

Chapter 8
Allergic Reactions/Ingestions

English	Spanish	Pronunciation
Are you hurt?	¿Está herido?	[ehs-tah air-ee-doe]
Where?	¿Dónde?	[don-day]
Show me.	Muéstreme.	[mwhe-stray may]
Did you faint?	¿Se desmayó?	[say des-my-oh]
Do you take any medications?	¿Toma medicinas?	[toe-mah meh-dee-see-nahs]
Get it.	Consíguelo.	[con-see-gay-low]
Can you sit up?	¿Puede sentarse?	[pway-day sen-tar-say]
Please lie down.	Acuéstese, por favor.	[ah-ques-tay-say poor fah-vore]

Allergic Reactions

Anaphylaxis

Are you allergic to...	¿Tiene alergias a...	[tee-eh-nay ah-lay-hee-ahs ah:]
Stings	Picaduras	[pee-cah-do-rahs]
Bees	Abejas	[ah-bay-hoss]
Wasps	Avispas	[ah-vees-pahs]
Hornets	Avispones	[ah-vees-pone-ehs]
Foods:	Comidas	[coe-mee-dahs]
Nuts	Nueces	[new-eh-says]
Fish	Pescado	[pes-cah-doe]
Shellfish (crabs, lobster)	Mariscos (cangrejo, langosta)	[mar-eez-coes con-gray-hoes, lane-ghost-ah]
Berries	Bayas	[bye-yahs]
Spices	Especias	[eh-speh-see-ahs]

Airborne substances

Pollen	Polen	*[poe-len]*
Dust	Polvo	*[pole-voe]*
Animal Hair	Pelo de los animales	*[pay-low day lows ah-nee-mah-lays]*
Chemicals	Químicos	*[key-me-coes]*
Do you take medication for allergies?	¿Toma medicina para alergias?	*[toe-mah meh-dee-see-nah par-ah ah-lare-hee-ahs]*

Ingested/Injected substances

Medicines	Medicinas	*[meh-dee-see-nahs]*
Penicillin	Penicilina	*[peh-nee-see-lee-nah]*
Tetracycline	Tetraciclina	*[tey-trah-see-clee-nah]*

ALLEGIY

Poisons   Venenos   *[veh-neh-knows]*

Ingested

What did you eat?	¿Qué comió?	*[kay coe-mee-oh]*
Foods	Comidas	*[coe-mee-das]*
Plants	Plantas	*[plan-tas]*
Medicines	Medicinas	*[meh-dee-see-nas]*
Cleaning Products	Quitamanchas	*[key-tah-mahn-chas]*
Household Poisons	Venenos caseros	*[veh-neh-knows cah-sare-rows]*
Rat Poison	Matarratas/ Ratacida	*[mat-ah-rat-ahs/rah-tah-see-dah]*

ALLERGY

Ingested

Fuels	Combustibles	
Gasoline	Gasolina	*[gah-so-lee-nah]*
Lighter Fluid	Fluida del encendedor	*[flu-ee-dah del en-sen-day-door]*
Kerosene	Kerosen	*[care-oh-sen]*

Injected   Inyectó

Stings	Picadura	*[pee-cah-do-rah]*
Spiders	Araña	*[ah-rahn-ya]*
Insects	Insecto	*[een-sek-toe]*
Snakes	Culebra	*[coo-lebb-rah]*
Needles	Aguja	*[ah-goo-hah]*

Inhaled   Aspiró

Cleaning Products	Quitamanchas	*[key-tah-mahn-chas]*
Household Poisons	Venenos caseros	*[veh-neh-knows cah-sare-rows]*
Exhaust Fumes	Humo del escape	*[oo-moe del eh-scah-pay]*

Absorbed   Absorbió

Cleaning Products	Quitamanchas	*[key-tah-mahn-chas]*

Chapter 9
Trauma

Are you hurt?	¿Está herido?	[ehs-tah air-ee-doe]
Where?	¿Dónde?	[don-day]
Show me.	Muéstreme.	[mwhe-stray may]
Did you faint?	¿Se desmayó?	[say des-my-oh]
Do you take any medications?	¿Toma medicinas?	[toe-mah meh-dee-see nahs]
Get it.	Consíguelo.	[con-see-gay-low]
Can you sit up?	¿Puede sentarse?	[pway-day sen-tar-say]
Please lie down.	Acuéstese, por favor.	[ah-ques-tay-say poor fah-vore]

Trauma

Does your head hurt?	¿Le duele su cabeza?	[lay dwell-lay sue cah-bay-sah]
Do not move your head.	No se mueve su cabeza.	[no say mway-vay sue cah-bay-sah]
Does your neck hurt?	¿Le duele su cuello?	[lay dwell-lay sue kway-yo]
Do not move your neck.	No se mueve su cuello.	[no say mway-vay sue kway-yo]
Did you lose consciousness?	¿Perdió el conocimiento?	[pare-dee-oh el coe-no-see-me-ehn-toe]
For how long?	¿Por cuánto tiempo?	[pour kwahn-toe tee-ehm-poe]
Seconds?	¿Segundos?	[say-goon-dose]
Minutes?	¿Minutos?	[me-new-toes]
Hours?	¿Horas?	[ore-ahs]

Falls

Did you fall from...	¿Se cayó de...	*[say ky-yo day]*
Stairs	Escalera	*[es-cah-lare-ah]*
Ladder	Escalera portátil	*[es-cah-lare-ah poor-tah-teal]*
Roof	Tejado	*[tay-hah-doe]*
Window	Ventana	*[ven-tah-nah]*
Tree	Arbol	*[are-bowl]*
Chair	Silla	*[see-yah]*
Bike	Bicicleta	*[bee-see-cleh-tah]*

Motor Vehicle Accident

TRAUMA

Did you crash the car?	¿Chocó con un coche?	*[choe-coe con oon coe-chay]*
Did you use seatbelts?	¿Usó su citurón de seguridad?	*[ooh-sew sue see-too-ron day say-goo-ree-dad]*
Did you hit the windshield?	¿Le pegó el parabrisas?	*[lay pay-go el pah-rah-bree-sahs]*
Did you hit the steering wheel?	¿Le pegó el volante?	*[lay pay-go el voe-lahn-tay]*
What did you hit?	¿Chocó con que?	*[choe-coe con kay]*
Car	Coche	*[coe-chay]*
Tree	Arbol	*[are-bowl]*
Animal	Animal	*[ah-nee-mal]*
Did you lose consciousness?	¿Perdió el conocimiento?	*[pare-dee-oh el coe-no-see-me-ehn-toe]*
For how long?	¿Por cuánto tiempo?	*[pour kwahn-toe tee-ehm-poe]*
Seconds?	¿Segundos?	*[say-goon-dose]*
Minutes?	¿Minutos?	*[me-new-toes]*
Hours?	¿Horas?	*[ore-ahs]*

Fight	Pelea	*[Pay-lay-ah]*
Were you hit with a...	¿Golpió con que?	*[gol-pee-oh con kay]*
Bottle	Botella	*[bow-tay-yah]*
Knife	Cuchillo	*[coo-chee-yo]*
Bat	Bate	*[bah-tay]*
Kick	Puntapie	*[poon-tah-pee-ay]*
Fist	Puño	*[poon-yo]*

Gunshot	Escopeta	*[Ehs-coe-peh-tah]*
You were shot with a...	Le tiró con...	*[lay teer-oh con...]*
Handgun	Pistola	*[peace-toe-lah]*
Shotgun	Escopeta	*[es-coe-pet-ah]*
Rifle	Rifle	*[ree-flay]*
Bites	Mordidas	*[more-dee-dahs]*
What bit you?	¿Que le mordió?	*[kay lay more-dee-oh]*
Person	Persona	*[pare-sohn-ah]*
Dog	Perro	*[pare-oh]*
Cat	Gato	*[gah-toe]*
Rat	Rata	*[rah-tah]*

Chapter 10
Burns

English	Spanish	Pronunciation
Are you hurt?	¿Está herido?	[ehs-tah air-ee-doe]
Where?	¿Dónde?	[don-day]
Show me.	Muéstreme.	[mwhe-stray may]
Did you faint?	¿Se desmayó?	[say des-my-oh]
Do you take any medications?	¿Toma medicinas?	[toe-mah meh-dee-see-nahs]
Get it.	Consíguelo.	[con-see-gay-low]
Can you sit up?	¿Puede sentarse?	[pway-day sen-tar-say]
Please lie down.	Acuéstese, por favor.	[ah-ques-tay-say poor fah-vore]

Burns   Quemaduras   *[Kay-mah-do-rahs]*

How were you burned?	¿Como le quemó?	[coe-moe lay kay-moe]

Thermal

English	Spanish	Pronunciation
Fire/Flame	Fuego	[fway-go]
Steam	Vapor	[bah-poor]
Hot Liquid	Liquido caliente	[lee-key-doe cah-lee-ehn-tay]
Water	Agua	[ah-gwah]
Coffee	Café	[cah-fay]
Soup	Sopa	[so-pah]

Thermal

Hot Object	Objeto caliente	*[ohb-heh-toe cah-lee-ehn-tay]*
Stove	Hornilla	*[or-knee-ah]*
Oven	Horno	*[or-no]*
Iron	Plancha	*[plahn-cha]*
Car	Coche	*[coe-chay]*

Electrical   Electricidad   *[Ee-leck-tree-see-dad]*

Wires	Alambres electricos	*[ah-lahm-brace eh-leck-tree-coes]*
Outlet	Toma de corriente	*[toe-mah day core-ree-ehn-tay]*
Appliances	Aparatos electricos	*[ah-pah-rah-toes eh-leck-tree-coes]*
Lightning	Relampagos	*[ray-lam-pah-goes]*
Pathway:	Senda:	*[sen-dah]:*
Entrance/ Exit	Entrada/Salida	*[en-tra-dah/sa-lee-dah]*
Chemical	Químicos	*[key-mee-coes]*
Acid	Ácido	*[ah-see-doe]*
Lye	Lejía	*[lay-hee-ah]*
Bleach	Cloro	*[clor-oh]*
Cleaning Fluid	Quitamanchas	*[key-tah-mahn-chas]*
Gasoline	Gasolina	*[ga-so-lee-nah]*
Dry Ice	Carbohielo	*[car-boe-ee-yellow]*

BURNS

Chapter 11
Environmental Emergencies

Are you hurt?	¿Está herido?	[ehs-tah air-ee-doe]
Where?	¿Dónde?	[don-day]
Show me.	Muéstreme.	[mwhe-stray may]
Did you faint?	¿Se desmayó?	[say des-my-oh]
Do you take any medications?	¿Toma medicinas?	[toe-mah meh-dee-see-nahs]
Get it.	Consíguelo.	[con-see-gay-low]
Can you sit up?	¿Puede sentarse?	[pway-day sen-tar-say]
Please lie down.	Acuéstese, por favor.	[ah-ques-tay-say poor fah-vore]

Heat Emergencies

Were you outside?	¿Estuvo afuera?	[ehs-too-voe ah-fway-rah]
Working	¿Trabajando?	[trah- bah-han-doe]
Excercising?	¿Haciendo?	[ah-see-en-doe]
Were you inside the...	¿Estuvo adentro...	[ehs-too- voe ah-den-tro]
house without air conditioning?	la casa sin aire?	[la cah-sah seen aye-ray]
car without air conditioning?	el coche sin aire?	[el coe-chay seen aye-ray]
Were the windows down?	Ventanas abiertas?	[ven-tah-nas ah-bee-air-tas]
Do you have muscle cramps?	¿Tiene calambres?	[tee-eh-nay cah-lahm-brays]
Do you feel weak/ dizzy?	¿Se siente debil/ mareado?	[say see-ehn-tay day-beal/ mah-ray-ah-doe]

Heat Emergencies

Have you...		
Fainted	¿Desmayó?	*[des-may-oh]*
Had nausea	¿Náusea?	*[now-say-ah]*
Vomiting	¿Vomitó?	*[voe-me-toe]*
Have you been drinking ...	¿Ha tomado...	*[ah toe-mah-doe...]*
Water	Agua	*[ah-gwah]*
Juice	Jugo	*[who-go]*
Soda Pop	Gaseosas	*[gah-say-oh-sahs]*
Alcohol	Alcohol	*[all-coe-hall]*

Cold Emergencies

How long have you been outside?	¿Por cuanto tiempo estuvo afuera? *[pour kwahn-toe tee-ehm-poe ehs-too-voe ah-fway-rah]*
An hour?	¿Una hora? *[ooh-nah ore-ah]*
Several hours?	¿Más de dos horas? *[moss day dose ore-ahs]*
More than eight hours?	¿Más de ocho horas? *[moss day oh-choe ore-ahs]*
All day/night?	¿Todo el día/noche? *[toe-doe el dee-ah/no-chay]*
Were you walking?	¿Estuvo caminando? *[ehs-too-voe cah-me-non-doe]*
Were you sitting/lying	¿Estuvo sentando/acostando? *[ehs-too-voe sen-tahn-doe/ah-coe-stahn-doe]*
Have you had any alcohol?	¿Tomó alcohól? *[toe-moe al-coe-hol]*

ENVIRONMENTAL

Water Related Emergencies

Near Drowning

Questions for bystanders with an unconcious patient

How long was he underwater?	¿Por cuánto tiempo estuvo él abajo el agua? *[pour kwahn-toe tee-ehm-poe ehs-too-voe el ah-bah-hoe el ah-gwah]*
1 minute	Un minuto *[oon me-new-toe]*
5 minute	Cinco minutos *[sink-oh me-new-toes]*
10 minutes	Diez minutos *[dee-ace me-new-toes]*
20 minutes	Veinte minutos *[vane-tay me-new-toes]*
More	Más *[moss]*
Unknown	No sabe *[no sah-bay]*

Questions for bystanders in a pool related injury

Did he dive into the pool?	¿Se zambulló en la piscina? *[say sam-boo-yoe en la pee-see-nah]*
from the diving board	de la plataforma *[day la pla-tah-for-mah]*
Did he/she hit his/her head on the board?	¿Chocó con la plataforma? *[choe-coe con la pla-tah-formah]*

Chapter 12
OB/GYN

Are you having contractions?	¿Tiene contracciónes? *[tee-eh-nay con-track-see-own-ehs]*
Tell me when they start and stop.	¿Dígame cuando empiezan y paran. *[dee-gah-may kwahn-doe ehm-pee-ay-son eee pah-ron]*
Do you have to push?	¿Tiene que empujar? *[tee-eh-nay kay ehm-poo-har]*
Has your water broken?	¿Se le reventó la fuente? *[say lay ray-ven-toe la fwen-tay]*

Gynecology

Are you having non-menstrual vaginal bleeding?	¿Está sangrando de la vagina y no es su regla? *[es-tah sahn-grahn-doe day la vah-hee-nah eee no es sue re-glah]*
Are you pregnant?	¿Está embarazada? *[es-tah em-bah-rah-sah-dah]*

Childbirth — Alumbramiento

Are you pregnant?	¿Está embarazada? *[eh-stah ehm-bar-ah-sah-dah]*
How many months? (show fingers)	¿Cuántos meses? *[kwahn-toes may-says]*
Is this your first child?	¿Es su primer niño? *[ehs sue pre-mare-oh neen-yo]*

Childbirth	Alumbramiento

How many pregnancies have you had?
¿Cuántos embarazos ha tenido?
[kwahn-toes ehm-bah-rah-sews ah teh-nee-doe]

Have you seen a doctor since you have been pregnant?
¿Ha visitado el médico desde que ha estado embarazada?
[ah vee-see-tah-doe el may-dee-coe dez-day kay ah eh-tah-do ehm-bah-rah-sah-dah]

Did you have a C-section?
¿Tuvó un cesárea?
[too-voe oon say-sah-ray-ah]

How long have you had labor pains?
¿Por cuánto tiempo ha tenido dolores del parto?
[pour kwahn-toe tee-ehm-poe ah teh-nee-doe doe-lore-rays del par-toe]

Has your water broken?
¿Se le reventó la fuente?
[say lay ray-ven-toe la fwen-tay]

Was it ...?
¿Era ...   *[air-ah...]*

clear   clara   *[clah-rah]*

red   roja   *[roe-hah]*

yellow   amarilla   *[ah-mah-ree-yah]*

green   verde   *[vare-day]*

Do you have to push?
¿Necessita empujar?
[nay-say-see-tah ehm-poo-har]

Do you feel like you need to move your bowels?
¿Necessita hacer poo-poo?
[nay-say-see-tah ah-sare poo-poo]

Pre-Eclampsia/Supine

Hypertensive Syndrome

Are you dizzy?	¿Está vertiginosa?
	[eh-stah vare-tee-heen-oh-sah]
Lie on your left side.	Acuéstese en su lado izquierdo.
	[ah-ques-tay-say en sue lah-do ease-key-air-doe]

Excessive Bleeding

Are you bleeding a lot?	¿Está sangrando mucho?
	[eh-stah sahn-grahn-doe moo-choe]
Lie on your left side.	Acuéstese en su lado izquierdo.
	[ah-ques-tay-say en sue lah-do ease-key-air-doe]

Injuries to a pregnant patient

Have you fallen?	¿Se cayó?
	[say kai-yo]
[see "Falls" in the Trauma section for appropriate questions.]	
Are you having cramps?	¿Teine calambres?
	[tee-eh-nay cah-lahm-brace]
How many months pregnant are you?	¿Cuántos meses está embarazada?
	[kwahn-toes may-says eh-stah ehm-bah rah-sah-dah]

OB/GYN

Delivery	Parto	
Lie down.	Acuéstese. *[ah-ques-tay-say]*	
Bring your knees up.	Traiga sus rodillas arriba. *[try-gah soos roe-dee-yas ah-ree-bah]*	
We are going to put a blanket under you.	Vamos a poner una blanketa debajo sus nalgas. *[vah-moes ah pone-air oo-nah blanket-ah day-bah-hoe soos nal-gahs]*	
Be calm.	Tranquila. *[tran-key-lah]*	
Relax.	Relájese.. *[ray-lah-hey-say]*	
Breathe through your mouth.	Respire con su boca. *[ray-spee-ray con sue boe-cah]*	

Push!	¡Empuje!	*[ehm-poo-hay]*
One	Uno	*[ew-no]*
Two	Dos	*[dose]*
Three	Tres	*[trace]*
Four	Cuatro	*[kwah-troe]*
Five	Cinco	*[sink-oh]*
Six	Seis	*[sace]*
Seven	Siete	*[see-eh-tay]*
Eight	Ocho	*[oh-choe]*
Nine	Nueve	*[new-ay-vay]*
Ten	Diez	*[dee-ace]*
Again.	Otra vez.	*[oh-trah vase]*
Don't Push!	¡No empuje!	*[no ehm-poo-hay]*
It's a boy/girl!	¡Es un varón/una niña!	*[ehs oon var-own/oo-nah neen-ya]*

Post-Birth

You may feel more contractions.	Es possible se siente mas contracciónes. *[ehs poe-see-blay say see-ehn-tay moss con-trah-see-oh-nays]*
These are normal.	Son normales. *[son nor-mah-lays]*

Chapter 13

Pediatrics

Are you hurt?	¿Está herido?	[ehs-tah air-ee-doe]
Where?	¿Dónde?	[don-day]
Show me.	Muéstreme.	[mwhe-stray may]
Did you faint?	¿Se desmayó?	[say des-my-oh]
Do you take any medications?	¿Toma medicinas?	[toe-mah meh-dee-see nahs]
Get it.	Conséguelo.	[con-see-gay-low]
Can you sit up?	¿Puede sentarse?	[pway-day sen-tar-say]
Please lie down.	Acuéstese, por favor.	[ah-ques-tay-say poor fah-vore]

Infants and Young Children (Patients)

Questions for parents/guardians

What is his/her name?	¿Cómo se llama?	[coe-moe say yah-mah]
How old is he/she?	¿Cuántos años (years) /meses (months) tiene?	[kwahn-toes ahn-yoes/ may-says tee-eh-nay]
How much does he/she weigh?	¿Cuánto pesa?	[kwahn-toe peh-sah]
Is he/she sick?	¿Está enfermo(a)?	[eh-stah ehn-fair moe (mah)]
Did he/she...?		
vomit	¿Vomitó?	[voe-me-toe]
have diarrhea	¿Tiene diarrea?	[tee-eh-nay dee-ah-ray-ah]
have a cough	¿Tiene tos?	[tee-eh-nay tose]

Infants and Young Children (Patients)

have a fever	¿Tiene fiebre?	[tee-eh-nay fee-eh-bray]
For how long?	¿Por cuánto tiempo?	[pour kwahn-toe tee-ehm-poe]
Hours	Horas?	[ore-ahs]
Days?	Días?	[dee-ahs]
have seizures?	¿Tiene convul-siones?	[tee-eh-nay cone-vool-see-oh-nase]
How many?	¿Cuántos?	[kwahn-toes]
Did you give him/her medicine ?	¿Le dió medicina?	[lay dee-oh may-dee-see-nah]
What medicine?	Qué medicina?	[kay may-dee-see-nah]
Show me.	Muéstreme.	[mwhe-stray may]
Is he/she hurt?	¿Le duele?	[lay dwell-lay]
Where?	¿Dónde?	[don-day]
Show me.	Muéstreme.	[mwhe-stray may]
Was this an accident?	¿Era un accidente?	[air-ah oon ack-see-den-tay]
Did someone hurt him/her?	¿Alguien le duele?	[al-gee-ehn lay dwell-lay]
Who?	¿Quién?	[key-ehn]

For patient assessment, use appropriate section of manual to guide your questioning.

Older Children

Questions for child patient

My name is _____.	Me llamo _____. [may yah-moe_____]
We are going to help.	Vamos a ayudarle. [vah-moes ah aye-you-dar-lay]

PEDIATRICS

Older Children

What is your name?	Cómo se llama?
	[coe-moe say yah-mah]
How old are you?	Cuántos años tiene?
	[kwahn-toes ahn-yoes tee-eh-nay]
Are your parents here?	Sus padres están aquí?
	[soos pah-drays eh-stahn ah-key]
Where do you live?	Dónde vive?
	[don-day vee-vay]
What is the address?	¿La dirección?
	[la dee-wreck-see-own]
What is the phone number?	¿El número de teléfono?
	[el New-mare-oh day teh-lay-foe-no]
Are you sick?	¿Está enfermo?
	[eh-stah en-fare-moe]
Where?	¿Dónde? *[don-day]*
Are you hurt?	¿Está herido? *[eh-stah air-ee-doe]*
Where?	¿Dónde? *[don-day]*
Show me.	Muéstreme. *[mwhe-stray may]*
Was this an accident?	¿Fue un accidente?
	[fway oon ack-see-den-tay]
Did someone hurt you?	¿Alguien le duele?
	[al-gee-ehn lay dwell-lay]
Who?	¿Quién? *[key-ehn]*
I need to move your clothes so can listen to your...	Necessito mover su ropa para escuchar a isu...
	[neh-she-see-toe moe-vare sue row-pah pah-rah es-coo-char ah sue...]
Heart	Corazón *[core-ah-zone]*
Lungs	Pulmones *[pool-moan-ehs]*

To further assess patient, use appropriate sections of this manual to guide your questions

For agencies that carry stuffed animals for pediatric patients.

Look, a stuffed animal for you.	¡Mira, un juguete para ti! *[me-rah oon who-geh-tay pah-rah tee]*
What is his name?	¿Cómo se llama? *[coe-moe say yah-mah]*
That's a good name!	¡Es un nombre bonito! *[ehs oon nome-bray boe-nee-toe]*

Children with Parents Who Are Patients

My name is_____.	Me llamo _____. *[may yah-moe_____]*
We are here to help your father/mother.	Estamos aquí para ayudar su papá/mamá. *[eh-stah-moes ah-key pah-rah eye-you-dar sue papa/mama]*
What is your name?	¿Como se llama ustéd? *[coe-moe say yah-mah oo-sted]*
What is your parent's name?	¿Como se llama su mamá/papá? *[coe-moe say yah-mah sue mama/papa]*
How old is your mother/father?	¿Cuántos años tiene su mamá/papá? *[kwahn-toes ahn-yoes tee-eh-nay sue mama/papa]*

To further assess patient, use appropriate section of this manual to guide your questions.

PEDIATRICS

Chapter 14
Patient Transport and Refusals

Are you hurt?	¿Está herido?	[ehs-tah air-ee-doe]
Where?	¿Dónde?	[don-day]
Show me.	Muéstreme.	[mwhe-stray may]
Did you faint?	¿Se desmayó?	[say des-my-oh]
Do you take any medications?	¿Toma medicinas?	[toe-mah meh-dee-see nahs]
Get it.	Consíguelo.	[con-see-gay-low]
Can you sit up?	¿Puede sentarse?	[pway-day sen-tar-say]
Please lie down.	Acuéstese, por favor.	[ah-ques-tay-say poor fah-vore]

Transport

Do you want to go to the hospital?	¿Quiere ir al hospital? [key-air-ray ear all hos-pee-tal]
You need to go to the hospital.	Necessita ir al hospital. [neh-say-see-toe ear al hos-pee-tal]
You do not need to go to the hospital.	No necessita ir al hospital. [no neh-say-see-toe ear al hos-pee-tal]
We are going to take you to the hospital.	Vamos a llevarle al hospital. [vah-moes ah yay-var-lay a hos-pee-tal]
The name of the hospital is _____.	El nombre del hospital es _____. [el nome-bray del hos-pee-tal ehs____.]
We are going to take you to the hospital by helicopter.	Vamos a hospital por helicoptero. [vah-moes ah hos-pee-tal pour heh-lee-cop-tare-oh]

Refusals

For cases when the patient should go to the hospital but does not want to.

You need to go to the hospital.

Necessita ir al hospital.
[neh-say-see-tah ear al hos-pee-tal]

We cannot force you to go, but you should.

No podemos a forsarle pero debería ir.
[no poe-deh-moes ah four-sar-lay, pare-oh deh-bare-ree-ah ear.]

You can change your mind and we can take you.

Puede cambiar su mente y podemos llevarle.
[pway-day cam-bee-are sue men-tay ee poe-deh-moes yay-var-lay]

For ordinary refusals

This form says that you do not want to go to the hospital. Sign here.

Este papel dice no quiere ir al hospital.
[eh-stay pah-pel dee-say no key-air-ray ear al hos-pee-tal]

Firme aquí.
[fear-may ah-kay]

TRANSPORT/REFUSAL

Chapter 15
Fire Calls

Is anyone hurt?	¿Alguien tiene daños?	[al-gui-ehn tee-eh-nay dawn-yoes]
Is everyone out of the house?	¿Todos están afuera?	[toe-does eh-stahn ah-fway-rah]
How many people are inside	¿Cuántas personas están adentro?	[kwahn-toes pare-so-nahs eh-stahn ah-den-tro]
One	Uno	[ew-no]
Two	Dos	[dose]
Three	Tres	[trace]
More than four	Más que cuatro	[mahs kay kwah-troe]
Are they in the...	¿Están en el...?	[eh-stahn en el...]
Bedroom	Cuarto de dormir	[kwar-toe day door-meer]
Front of house	En el frente	[en el fren-tay]
Back of house	Detrás	[day-tross]
Bathroom	Baño	[bahn-yo]
Front of house	En el frente	[en el fren-tay]
Back of house	Detrás	[day-tross]
Basement	Sótano	[so-tah-no]
Is the fire in the ...	¿El fuego está en... ?	[el fway-go eh-stah en...]
Kitchen	Cocina	[coe-see-nah]
Laundry	Lavanderia	[lay-vahn-dah-ree-ah]
Basement	Sótano	[so-tah-no]
Bedroom	Cuarto de dormir	[kwar-toe day door-meer]
Upstairs	Arriba	[ah-ree-bah]
Downstairs	Abajo	[ah-bah-hoe]
Bathroom	Baño	[bahn-yo]
Upstairs	Arriba	[ah-ree-bah]
Downstairs	Abajo	[ah-bah-hoe]

Where is the room?	¿Donde está el cuarto?	[don-day ehs-tah el kwar-toe]
Show me the room.	Muéstreme el cuarto.	[mweh-stray-may el kwar-toe]
Is everyone out now?	¿Todos están afuera ahora?	[toe-dose eh-stahn ah-fway-rah ah-ore-ah]
You cannot go back inside!	¡No puede regresar adentro!	[no pway-day ray-greh-sar ah-den-tro]

Appendix A
Additional Anatomical Illustrations

Skeleton/Esqueleto
Anterior View/Vista Anterior

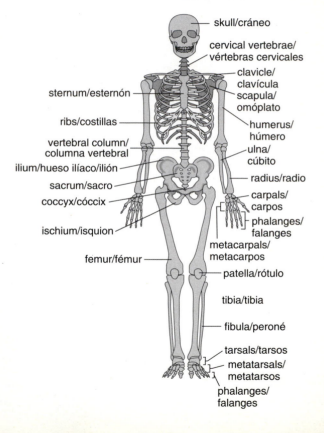

skull/cráneo

cervical vertebrae/
vértebras cervicales

clavicle/
clavícula

scapula/
omóplato

sternum/esternón

humerus/
húmero

ribs/costillas

vertebral column/
columna vertebral

ulna/
cúbito

ilium/hueso ilíaco/ilión

radius/radio

sacrum/sacro

carpals/
carpos

coccyx/cóccix

phalanges/
falanges

ischium/isquion

metacarpals/
metacarpos

femur/fémur

patella/rótulo

tibia/tibia

fibula/peroné

tarsals/tarsos

metatarsals/
metatarsos

phalanges/
falanges

Skeleton/Esqueleto
Posterior View/Vista Posterior

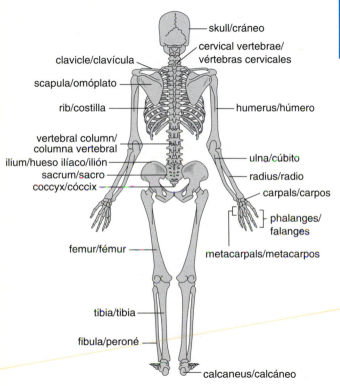

skull/cráneo

cervical vertebrae/
vértebras cervicales

clavicle/clavícula

scapula/omóplato

rib/costilla

humerus/húmero

vertebral column/
columna vertebral

ilium/hueso ilíaco/ilión

sacrum/sacro

coccyx/cóccix

ulna/cúbito

radius/radio

carpals/carpos

phalanges/
falanges

femur/fémur

metacarpals/metacarpos

tibia/tibia

fibula/peroné

calcaneus/calcáneo

Structures of the Eye
Estructuras del Ojo

Lateral View of the Eyeball Interior
Vista Lateral del Globo del Ojo Interior

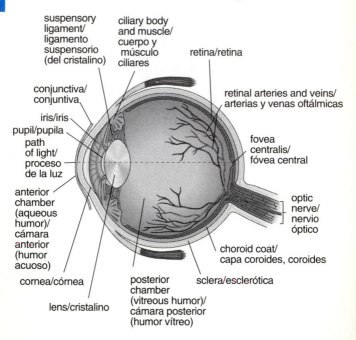

suspensory ligament/ ligamento suspensorio (del cristalino)

ciliary body and muscle/ cuerpo y músculo ciliares

retina/retina

conjunctiva/ conjuntiva

retinal arteries and veins/ arterias y venas oftálmicas

iris/iris

pupil/pupila

path of light/ proceso de la luz

fovea centralis/ fóvea central

anterior chamber (aqueous humor)/ cámara anterior (humor acuoso)

optic nerve/ nervio óptico

cornea/córnea

choroid coat/ capa coroides, coroides

lens/cristalino

posterior chamber (vitreous humor)/ cámara posterior (humor vítreo)

sclera/esclerótica

Structures of the Ear
Estructuras del Oído

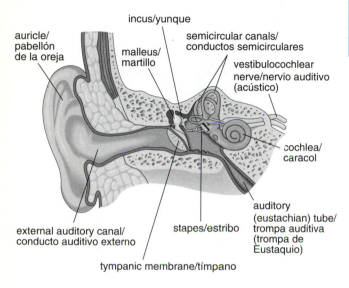

incus/yunque

auricle/
pabellón
de la oreja

malleus/
martillo

semicircular canals/
conductos semicirculares

vestibulocochlear
nerve/nervio auditivo
(acústico)

cochlea/
caracol

external auditory canal/
conducto auditivo externo

stapes/estribo

auditory
(eustachian) tube/
trompa auditiva
(trompa de
Eustaquio)

tympanic membrane/tímpano

Structures of the Mouth
Estructuras del la Boca

epiglottis/epiglotis

right palatine tonsil/ amígdala palatina derecha

left palatine tonsil/ amígdala palatina izquierda

lingual tonsil/ amígdala lingual

wisdom tooth/ muela del juicio

gum/encía

molars/ molares

tongue/lengua

bicuspids/ bicúspides o premolares

cuspid/canino

lateral incisor/ incisivo lateral

central incisor/incisivo central

Digestive System
Aparato o Sistema Digestivo

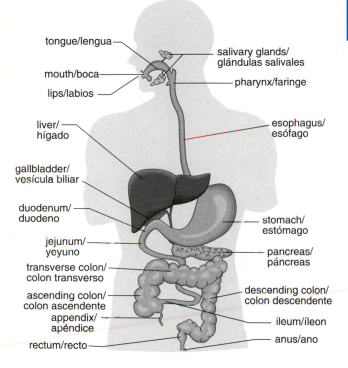

tongue/lengua

mouth/boca

lips/labios

salivary glands/
glándulas salivales

pharynx/faringe

liver/
hígado

esophagus/
esófago

gallbladder/
vesícula biliar

duodenum/
duodeno

stomach/
estómago

jejunum/
yeyuno

pancreas/
páncreas

transverse colon/
colon transverso

ascending colon/
colon ascendente

descending colon/
colon descendente

appendix/
apéndice

ileum/íleon

rectum/recto

anus/ano

Respiratory System
Aparato o Sistema Respiratorio

sphenoid sinus/seno esfenoidal

nasopharynx/nasofaringe

oropharynx/orofaringe

laryngopharynx/
laringofaringe

esophagus/esófago

right lung/
pulmón derecho

right bronchus/
bronquio derecho

terminal bronchioles/
bronquíolos terminales

alveoli/alvéolos

frontal sinus/seno frontal

nasal cavity/fosa nasal

nose/nariz

chin/mentón o barbilla

epiglottis/epiglotis

larynx/laringe

trachea/tráquea

left lung/
pulmón
izquierdo

mediastinum/
mediastino

diaphragm/
diafragma

General or Systemic Circulation
Circulación General o Sistemática

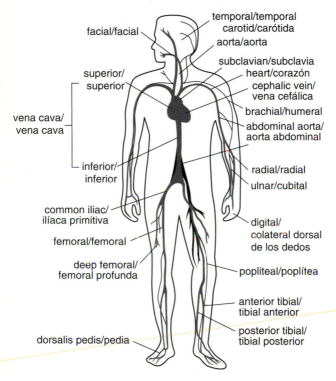

temporal/temporal
carotid/carótida

facial/facial

aorta/aorta

subclavian/subclavia
heart/corazón

superior/
superior

cephalic vein/
vena cefálica

brachial/humeral

vena cava/
vena cava

abdominal aorta/
aorta abdominal

inferior/
inferior

radial/radial

ulnar/cubital

common iliac/
ilíaca primitiva

digital/
colateral dorsal
de los dedos

femoral/femoral

deep femoral/
femoral profunda

popliteal/poplítea

anterior tibial/
tibial anterior

posterior tibial/
tibial posterior

dorsalis pedis/pedia

Urinary System
Sistema Urinario o Aparato Urinario

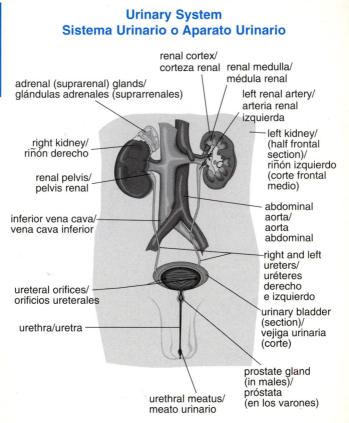

renal cortex/
corteza renal

renal medulla/
médula renal

adrenal (suprarenal) glands/
glándulas adrenales (suprarrenales)

left renal artery/
arteria renal
izquierda

right kidney/
riñón derecho

left kidney/
(half frontal
section)/
riñón izquierdo
(corte frontal
medio)

renal pelvis/
pelvis renal

inferior vena cava/
vena cava inferior

abdominal
aorta/
aorta
abdominal

right and left
ureters/
uréteres
derecho
e izquierdo

ureteral orifices/
orificios ureterales

urinary bladder
(section)/
vejiga urinaria
(corte)

urethra/uretra

prostate gland
(in males)/
próstata
(en los varones)

urethral meatus/
meato urinario

Appendix B

Additional Vocabulary Terms, English/Spanish

abandonment	abandono	*[ah-bahn-doe-noe]*
abrasion	escoración	*[ess-coh-rah-see-own]*
altered mental state	estado mental alterado	*[ess-tah-doe men-tahl all-tehr-ah-doe]*
anatomy	anatomía	*[ah-nah-toe-mee-ah]*
aorta	aorta	*[ah-oar-tah]*
artificial ventilation	respiración artificial	*[ress-pee-rah-see-own ahr-tee-fee-see-ahl]*
ausculate	escuchar	*[ess-coo-char]*
bandage	venda	*[ben-dah]*
blood vessel	vaso sanguíneo	*[bah-so san-guee-nay-oh]*
breach of confiden- tiality	abuso de cofianza	*[ah-boo-soe day don-fee- ahn-sah]*
burn	quemadura	*[kay-mah-doo-rah]*
cardiopulmonary resuscitation (CPR)	resucitación cardiopulmonar	*[ray-soo-see-tah-see-own car-de-oh-pool-moan- ahr]*
circulation	circulación	*[seer-coo-lah-see-own]*
confidentiality	confidentialidad	*[cone-fee-den-tee-ahl-ee- dahd]*
contusion	contusión	*[cone-two-see-own]*
cranium	cráneo	*[crah-nay-oh]*
cravat	pañuelo	*[pah-nyoo-eh-low]*
deformity	deformidad	*[day-for-mee-dahd]*
direct pressure	presión directo	*[preh-see-own dee-wreck- toe]*
dislocation	dislocación	*[dis-low-cah-see-own]*

dorsal	dorsal	*[door-sahl]*
dressing	vendaje;	*[ben-dah-hay]*;
	apósito	*[ah-poe-see-toe]*
embolism	embolia	*[ehm-bow-lee-ah]*
endocrine system	systema endocrino	*[sis-tehm-ah ehn-doe-cree-noe]*
epidermis	epidermis	*[eh-pee-dehr-mees]*
esophagus	esófago	*[eh-sew-fah-go]*
exhalation	espiración	*[ess-pee-rah-see-own]*
express consent	expresar consentimient; dar consentimiento	*[ex-press-ahr cohn-sent-oee-mee-ehn-toe]*; *[dahr cohn-sent-ee-mee-ehn-toe]*
femur	fémur	*[fay-mur]*
fibula	peroné	*[pay-row-nay]*
first responders	respondadores primeros	*[ray-spone-day-door-ace pree-may-rows]*
fracture	fractura	*[frack-two-rah]*
gag reflex	instinto de amordazar	*[een-steen-toe day ah-more-dah-zahr]*
gauze	malla	*[my-ah]*
glucose	glucosa	*[glue-coe-sah]*
Good Samaritan Laws	leyes de buenos samaritanos	*[lay-ace day boo-ay-nohs sah-mah-ree-tah-nohs]*
guarding	guardando; evitando	*[goo-are-dahn-doe]*; *[ay-bee-than-doe]*
hematoma	hematoma	*[ay-mah-toe-mah]*
hemorrhage	hemorragia	*[ay-more-ah-hee-ah]*
humerus	húmero	*[oo-mare-oh]*
hyperglycemia	hiperglucemia	*[ee-pair-glue-say-mee-ah]*
hypertension	hipertensión	*[ee-pair-ten-see-own]*
hyperthermia	hipertermia	*[ee-pair-tare-mee-ah]*

hyperventilate	hiperventilarse	*[ee-pair-ben-tee-lahr-say]*
hyperventilation	hiperventilación	*[ee-pair-ben-tee-lah-see-own]*
hypoglycemia	hipoglucemia	*[ee-poe-glue-seh-mee-ah]*
hypothermia	hipotermia	*[ee-poe-tare-mee-ah]*
hypoventilation	hipoventilación	*[ee-poe-ben-tee-lah-see-own]*
infection control	prevención de infección	*[pray-ben-see-own day-een-feck-see-own]*
inferior	inferior	*[een-fay-ree-or]*
initial assessment	evaluación principal	*[ee-bal-you-ah-see-own preen-see-pahl]*
laceration	laceración	*[lah-sare-ah-see-own]*
large intestine	intestino grueso	*[een-tes-teen-oh grew-ay-so]*
larynx	laringe	*[lah-reen-hay]*
lateral	lateral	*[lah-tare-ahl]*
ligament	ligamento	*[lee-gah-men-toe]*
liver	hígado	*[ee-gah-doe]*
lumbar vertebrae	vertebras lumbares	*[bare-tay-brahs loom-bar-ace]*
mandible	mandíbula	*[mahn-dee-boo-lah]*
maxilla	maxilar	*[mah-hee-lahr]*
negligence	negligencia	*[nay-glee-hen-see-ah]*
neonate	recién nacido	*[ray-see-ehn nah-see-doe]*
nervous system	systema nerviosa	*[sis-tehm-ah nare-vee-of-sah]*
pallor	palidez	*[pah-lee-daze]*
pancreas	páncreas	*[pahn-cray-ahs]*
paradoxical motion	movimiento paradójico	*[moe-bee-mee-ehn-toe pah-rah-doe-hee-coe]*
paralysis	parálisis	*[pah-rah-lee-sees]*
pharynx	faringe	*[fah-reen-hay]*
posterior	trasero	*[trah-sare-oh]*

postural hypoten-sion	hypotension postural	*[ee-poe-ten-see-own pohs-two-rahl]*
pressure dressing	vendaje de presión	*[ben-dah-hay day pray-see-own]*
pressure points	puntos de presión	*[poon-toes day pray-see-own]*
pulse	pulso	*[pool-so]*
pupil	pupila	*[poo-peel-ah]*
raccoon's eyes	ojos de mapache	*[oh-hoes day mah-pay-chay]*
rapid trauma assessment	evaluación rapida de trauma	*[ay-bahl-you-ah-see-own rah-pee-dah day trow-mah]*
resuscitate	resucitar	*[ray-soo-see-tar]*
Ryan White Law	ley de Ryan White	*[lay day Ryan White]*
scene survey	evaluación de la escena	*[ay-bahl-you-ah-see-own day lah eh-say-nah]*
seizure	ataque	*[ah-tah-kay]*
size-up	evaluar	*[ay-bahl-you-are]*
sling and swathe (S/S)	cabestrillar y envolver	*[cah-bay-stree-yar ee ehn-vole-vare]*
small intestine	intestine delgago	*[een-tess-teen-oh dell-gah-doe]*
superficial	superficial	*[soo-pare-fee-see-ahl]*
superior (toward or on the top of)	encima de	*[ehn-see-mah day]*
tachycardia	taquicardia	*[tah-key-car-dee-ah]*
tendon	tendón	*[ten-done]*
thoracic vertebrae	vertebras torácicas	*[bare-tayt-brahs tore-ah-see-kahs]*
traction	tracción	*[track-see-own]*

ulna	cúbito	*[coo-bee-toe]*
unresponsive	insensible;	*[een-sehn-see-blay]*;
	que no responde	*[kay no ray-spon-day]*
urticaria	urticaria	*[oor-tee-car-ee-ah]*
wound	herida	*[air-ee-dah]*